COMPLETE GUIDE TO UNDERSTANDING KNEE REPLACEMENT SURGERY

A Detailed Manual On Procedures, Recovery, Risks, Alternatives For Arthritis Relief And Joint Health Improvement

KLEIN HOYLE

Disclaimer

The content in this book is based on the author's expertise and comprehension of the topic. The author has no affiliation or link with any corporation, business, or person. This book is meant to give general information and educational material only, and it should not be interpreted as professional medical advice. Always seek the advice of a skilled healthcare expert if you have any queries about medical issues or treatments. The author and publisher expressly disclaim any responsibility resulting directly or indirectly from the use or use of the information included in this book.

Table of Contents

CHAPTER 1 15

Introduction To Knee Replacement Surgery 15

What Is A Knee Replacement Surgery? 15

When Is Knee Replacement Surgery Necessary? .16

1. Severe osteoarthritis: 16

3. Post-traumatic arthritis: 17

4. Other conditions: 17

Overview Of Knee Anatomy 17

Brief History Of Knee Replacement Surgery 18

CHAPTER 2 21

Understanding Knee Problems 21

Common Knee Problems That Lead To Surgery .21

Symptoms Of Knee Conditions 22

Diagnostic Procedures 23

Nonsurgical Treatment Options 24

3. Weight Management: 25

4. Assistive Devices: 25

5. Lifestyle Changes: 26

CHAPTER 3 27

Preparing For Knee Replacement Surgery 27

Consultation With An Orthopedic Surgeon 27

Pre-Operative Examinations And Assessments ..28

Physical Therapy And Exercise 30

Lifestyle Changes Before Surgery 31

CHAPTER 4 33

Types Of Knee Replacement Surgery 33

Total Knee Replacement (TKR) 33

Partial Knee Replacement (PKR) 34

Revision Knee Replacement.........................36

Minimally Invasive Knee Replacement Techniques

....37

CHAPTER 5 41

The Surgical 41

Anesthesia Options 41

1. General Anesthesia: 41

3. Mixture anesthetic: 42

Step-By-Step Overview Of Surgery 43

1. Preparation: 43

2. Incision:...43

3. Resection of Damaged Tissues: 43

4. Implant Placement: 44

5. Closure: 44

Duration Of Surgery 44

Potential Risks And Complications 45

1. Infection: 45

2. Blood Clots: 46

3. Implant Problems: 46

4. Nerve or Blood Vessel Damage: 46

5. Allergic Reactions or Anesthesia difficulties:

....46

CHAPTER 6 49

Recovery Process 49

The Hospital Stay After Surgery.................49

Pain Management Strategies 50

Physical Therapy And Rehabilitation Exercises..51

Expected Recovery Timeline 52

CHAPTER 7 55

Post-Op Care 55

Homecare Instructions 55

1. Activity Level:..55

2. Pain Management:...................................56

3. Mobility Aids: 56

4. Diet & Nutrition: 56

5. Follow-Up Appointments: 56

6. Home Environment:....................57

Wound Care 57

1. Keep the Incision Clean and Dry: 58

2. Change Dressings as Directed:..............58

3. Monitor for Infection: 58

4. Prevent Irritating the Incision: 59

5. Follow-Up Care: 59

Medication Management 60

1. Pain Management:.....................60

2. Antibiotics:.........................60

3. Blood Thinners: 61

4. Other drugs:........................61

5. Side Effects: 61

6. Medication Schedule: 62

Monitoring For Complications 62

1. Infection: 62

2. Blood Clots:........................63

3. Joint Stiffness or Instability:................63

4. Nerve Damage:......................64

CHAPTER 8 65

Lifestyle Modifications Following Surgery 65

Adaptive Equipment And Aids 65

Recommended Exercises To Strengthen The Knee
....66

Dietary Concerns For Optimal Recovery..........67

Return To Daily Activities And Work 68

CHAPTER 9 71

Possible Complications And Risks..................71

Blood Clots 72

Implant Failure 73

Nerve Or Blood Vessel Damage 75

CHAPTER 10 77

Long-Term Prospects And Follow-Up 77

Longevity Of Knee Implants 77

Monitoring For Signs Of Wear And Tear 78

Follow-Up Appointments With The Surgeon 80

Tips For Maintaining Knee Health After Surgery
....81

1. Follow Rehabilitation Guidelines: 81

2. Maintain a Healthy Weight:.....................82

3. Stay Active: 82

4. Avoid Overexertion: 82

5. Protect the Knee Joint: 83

Conclusion 84

THE END 87

ABOUT THIS BOOK

In the broad world of medical literature, the "Complete Guide to Understanding Knee Replacement Surgery" stands out as a light of clarity and direction for anyone navigating the complexity of knee health. From the first pages to the thorough investigation of post-operative care, this book is a reliable companion for patients, caregivers, and healthcare professionals alike.

Chapter 1 establishes the framework for knee replacement surgery by demystifying it, explaining why it is necessary, and offering a detailed grasp of knee anatomy. A succinct historical perspective provides readers with insight into the history of this surgical operation, creating a greater respect for its importance in contemporary healthcare.

Chapter 2 digs into the complex network of knee disorders, including prevalent conditions such as osteoarthritis and rheumatoid arthritis.

This part teaches readers how to spot the symptoms of knee problems and seek prompt treatment by going over diagnostic techniques. Furthermore, it emphasizes nonsurgical treatment options, providing a comprehensive approach to knee care.

Preparation is essential, and Chapter 3 walks readers through the pre-operative process in great detail. From consultations with orthopedic doctors to lifestyle changes, every detail is carefully considered, ensuring that clients begin on their surgical path completely educated and prepared.

In Chapter 4, this book delves into the many types of knee replacement surgery, including complete knee replacements and minimally invasive treatments. By explaining each procedure's complexities, readers get clarity on their alternatives, allowing them to make educated decisions in partnership with their healthcare practitioners.

Chapter 5 brings the operating theater to life, with detailed descriptions of anesthetic alternatives and procedural stages. By sharing light on possible risks and problems, this section helps patients prepare for surgery and gain confidence.

Chapter 6 takes readers on a journey of recovery, leading them through the postoperative terrain with compassion and skill. From pain management measures to rehabilitation activities, every aspect of healing is examined, encouraging hope and perseverance in patients.

Chapter 7 focuses on post-operative care, providing readers with extensive information on home care, wound management, and prescription regimes. By stressing attentiveness in monitoring for complications, this part promotes a culture of proactive healthcare involvement.

Chapter 8 marks the beginning of a new chapter in patients' lives, providing insights into lifestyle changes after surgery. From adaptive equipment to nutritional concerns, readers are equipped to maximize their recovery path and regain their quality of life.

Chapter 9 addresses potential obstacles and hazards front on, ensuring that readers are prepared to face challenges with resilience and educated decision-making. This part promotes a culture of vigilance and empowerment by raising awareness about infection, blood clots, and implant failure.

Finally, Chapter 10 looks forward to the long-term prognosis and follow-up, including tips on monitoring knee health and maintaining post-surgical well-being. This part, via longevity suggestions and follow-up sessions, ensures that patients start on a road to lifetime knee health with confidence and resilience.

In essence, the "Complete Guide to Understanding Knee Replacement Surgery" goes beyond the scope of a book, emerging as a beacon of hope, empowerment, and resilience in the landscape of knee health, leading readers through every step of their surgical journey with compassion and competence.

CHAPTER 1

Introduction To Knee Replacement Surgery

What Is A Knee Replacement Surgery?

Knee replacement surgery, also known as knee arthroplasty, is a medical operation that involves replacing damaged or worn-out elements of the knee joint with artificial materials. This procedure is often advised for those who have significant knee pain, stiffness, and limited mobility as a result of osteoarthritis, rheumatoid arthritis, or an accident.

During knee replacement surgery, damaged elements of the knee joint, such as the ends of the femur (thigh bone) and tibia (shinbone), are replaced with metal, plastic, or ceramic prosthetic components. These prosthetic components mirror the function of the native knee joint, allowing for more mobility and less discomfort.

When Is Knee Replacement Surgery Necessary?

Knee replacement surgery is often considered when alternative conservative therapies, such as medicines, physical therapy, and lifestyle changes, do not give significant relief for knee pain and mobility concerns. Common causes for knee replacement surgery include:

1. Severe osteoarthritis: Osteoarthritis is a degenerative joint condition in which cartilage breaks down in the knee joint. When conservative therapy is no longer effective in relieving the pain and stiffness associated with severe osteoarthritis, knee replacement surgery may be indicated.

2. Rheumatoid arthritis is an inflammatory illness that causes inflammation of the synovium (the joint's lining), resulting in cartilage destruction and joint deformity. In extreme situations, knee replacement surgery may be required to restore function and relieve discomfort.

3. Post-traumatic arthritis: Traumatic knee injuries, such as fractures or ligament tears, might increase the likelihood of developing arthritis over time. When these accidents cause severe joint damage and discomfort, knee replacement surgery may be the best way to restore mobility and function.

4. Other conditions: Knee replacement surgery may be indicated for people who have other knee joint problems, such as avascular necrosis (loss of blood flow to the bone), severe abnormalities, or prior knee operations that failed.

Overview Of Knee Anatomy

Grab knee replacement surgery requires a fundamental grasp of the anatomy of the knee joint. The knee is a complicated joint made up of three primary bones: the femur (thigh bone), the tibia (shinbone), and the patella. Ligaments, tendons, and cartilage link these bones, providing support and allowing the joint to move smoothly.

A coating of smooth, slippery cartilage covers the extremities of the femur and tibia, cushioning the bones and allowing them to slide easily against each other during movement. The patella sits in front of the knee joint and moves up and down in a groove in the femur when the knee bends and straightens.

The knee joint is surrounded by ligaments that provide stability and support, including the anterior ACL, PCL, MCL, and LCL are the four types of collateral ligaments. These ligaments act together to prevent excessive movement and keep the knee joint in good alignment.

Brief History Of Knee Replacement Surgery

The notion of knee replacement surgery goes back to the early twentieth century when doctors started investigating techniques to treat severe knee pain and dysfunction. The earliest reported efforts at knee replacement surgery used materials like ivory, wood, and rubber to replace injured knee joints, but these early surgeries were often ineffective and had high rates of complications.

It wasn't until the mid-twentieth century that considerable advances in materials and surgical methods made knee replacement surgeries more dependable and effective. In the 1960s and 1970s, pioneering surgeons such as Sir John Charnley and Gunston and Marmor pioneered the notion of complete knee replacement, which involves replacing both the femoral and tibial components of the knee with metal and plastic implants.

Since then, knee replacement surgery has been continuously refined and improved, with advances in implant design, surgical procedures, and rehabilitation protocols resulting in better results and longer-lasting artificial knee joints. Knee replacement surgery is now one of the most frequent orthopedic operations, relieving and restoring function to millions of people worldwide who suffer from terrible knee ailments.

CHAPTER 2

Understanding Knee Problems

Common Knee Problems That Lead To Surgery

Knee difficulties may arise from a variety of disorders, with osteoarthritis and rheumatoid arthritis being two of the most prevalent causes demanding knee replacement surgery. Osteoarthritis, sometimes known as "wear and tear arthritis," develops as the protective cartilage at the ends of bones deteriorates over time. This may cause discomfort, stiffness, edema, and limited movement in the knee. Rheumatoid arthritis, on the other hand, is an autoimmune illness in which the body's immune system incorrectly assaults the synovium, the lining of the membranes that surround the joints. Over time, this may cause joint injury, discomfort, inflammation, and deformity in the knee.

In addition to these two primary causes, post-traumatic arthritis (caused by previous knee injuries), avascular necrosis (loss of blood supply to the bone), and other inflammatory conditions can all contribute to serious knee problems that may necessitate surgery. Understanding the underlying cause of knee discomfort is critical in deciding the best treatment option, including whether knee replacement surgery is required.

Symptoms Of Knee Conditions

Recognizing the signs of knee disorders is critical for early detection and treatment. Common symptoms include discomfort, especially when bearing weight or moving the knee joint, stiffness or limited range of motion, swelling or soreness around the knee, a sense of instability or weakness in the knee, and, in rare cases, loud popping or grinding sounds when moving.

The degree and frequency of these symptoms vary according to the underlying cause of the knee disease.

For example, pain from osteoarthritis may intensify with exercise and lessen with rest, but pain from rheumatoid arthritis may be more chronic and accompanied by additional systemic symptoms such as tiredness and fever. It is critical not to dismiss chronic knee pain or discomfort, since early treatment may frequently help avoid additional damage and improve long-term results.

Diagnostic Procedures

Knee issues are normally diagnosed using a combination of clinical and imaging studies. X-rays are often used to see the bones of the knee joint and may aid in the diagnosis of osteoarthritis, bone spurs, and other structural problems. However, X-rays alone may not give sufficient information to accurately detect soft tissue injury or inflammation.

When more detailed imaging is required, magnetic resonance imaging (MRI) scans may be requested. MRI scans employ strong magnets and radio waves to provide comprehensive pictures of the soft tissues around the knee joint, including cartilage, ligaments, tendons, and muscles. This is especially beneficial for finding rips or inflammation in the ligaments or meniscus, as well as monitoring the general health of the joint.

In addition to imaging studies, blood tests may be used to detect inflammatory disorders like rheumatoid arthritis or to rule out other underlying medical problems that may be causing knee discomfort.

Nonsurgical Treatment Options

Before deciding on knee replacement surgery, many patients may look into non-surgical treatments for managing their knee pain and improving function. This may include:

1. Over-the-counter pain medications such as acetaminophen and nonsteroidal anti-inflammatory medicines (NSAIDs) may help lessen the discomfort

and inflammation caused by knee arthritis. In rare circumstances, corticosteroid injections may be advised to alleviate knee discomfort and swelling.

2. An organized physical therapy program may help increase the strength, flexibility, and range of motion of the knee joint. Therapeutic exercises, stretching methods, and manual therapy may be used to treat particular areas of weakness or dysfunction.

3. **Weight Management:** Excess body weight may put additional stress on the knee joint, aggravating arthritic symptoms and increasing the chance of serious joint damage. Maintaining a healthy weight with a balanced diet and regular exercise may help prevent knee strain and improve overall joint health.

4. **Assistive Devices:** Using braces, orthotics, or walking aids may help support the knee joint and relieve discomfort while doing weight-bearing activities. These devices may assist increase stability and lessen

the danger of falling, especially for those who have severe joint disease or weakness.

5. Lifestyle Changes: Making simple changes to daily activities and routines, such as avoiding high-impact activities, using proper body mechanics when lifting or bending, and taking rest breaks during extended periods of activity, can help alleviate symptoms and protect the knee joint from further damage.

Many individuals may successfully manage their knee discomfort without the need for knee replacement surgery by investigating these non-surgical therapy alternatives. However, for those with advanced arthritis or significant joint degeneration who have not responded to conservative therapy, knee replacement surgery may be the best option for restoring function and improving quality of life.

CHAPTER 3

Preparing For Knee Replacement Surgery

Consultation With An Orthopedic Surgeon

The first step before having knee replacement surgery is to arrange a consultation with an orthopedic physician. This first consultation is critical because it enables the surgeon to evaluate your condition and decide if knee replacement surgery is the best line of action for you. During the appointment, the surgeon will evaluate your medical history, do a physical examination of your knee, and request further tests such as X-rays or MRIs to better understand the amount of damage to your knee joint.

The consultation also provides a chance for you to ask any questions you may have about the operation. You may talk about the risks and advantages of knee replacement surgery, as well as what to anticipate throughout the recovery period. It is important to communicate openly and honestly with your surgeon about your worries and expectations so that they may personalize the treatment plan to match your specific requirements.

Following the consultation, the surgeon will collaborate with you to create a specific treatment plan, which may involve knee replacement surgery as well as alternative conservative therapies like physical therapy or medication. They will also give you information on how to prepare for surgery, including any pre-operative tests or assessments that could be required.

Pre-Operative Examinations And Assessments

Before having knee replacement surgery, you will need to go through several pre-operative tests and examinations to verify that you are in good enough health for the operation. These tests may include blood tests, a chest X-ray, an electrocardiogram (ECG), and a urinalysis. The goal of these tests is to evaluate your general health and discover any underlying medical issues that may raise your chances of complications after surgery.

In addition to these tests, you may meet with additional members of the surgical team, such as anesthesiologists or physical therapists, to discuss your unique requirements and concerns. This collaborative approach guarantees that all parts of your treatment are coordinated and maximized for the greatest results.

Depending on your medical history and risk factors, your surgeon may suggest additional pre-operative tests, such as a cardiac stress test, or a consultation with a specialist, such as a cardiologist or pulmonologist. These extra exams assist in further evaluating your surgical readiness and identify any possible concerns that must be addressed before starting.

Physical Therapy And Exercise

Physical therapy and exercise are essential in preparation for knee replacement surgery. In the weeks preceding the operation, your surgeon may propose a personalized workout regimen to help strengthen the muscles around your knee joint while also improving flexibility and range of motion.

Physical therapy exercises may involve low-impact activities like walking, swimming, or cycling, as well as specialized exercises for the muscles in your legs and knees. These exercises not only enhance the general function of your knee joint but also assist in speeding up the healing process after surgery.

In addition to physical therapy exercises, your surgeon may prescribe lifestyle changes like decreasing weight or stopping smoking to improve your general health and lower the chance of problems following surgery. By actively participating in your pre-operative care, you may assist in ensuring the greatest possible result after knee replacement surgery.

Lifestyle Changes Before Surgery

Making lifestyle changes before and after knee replacement surgery may significantly enhance your general health and well-being. One key change is to maintain a healthy weight. Excess weight may place additional strain on your knee joints, aggravating discomfort and making it more difficult for your body to recover after surgery. You may acquire and maintain a healthy weight by eating a well-balanced diet and exercising regularly, which can enhance the results of your knee replacement surgery.

Another significant lifestyle change is stopping smoking. Smoking may reduce blood flow and oxygen supply to tissues, slowing the healing process after surgery and increasing the chance of problems like infection. If you smoke, stopping before surgery may greatly lower your risks and enhance the outcome of your knee replacement.

Furthermore, it is essential to create realistic plans for living following surgery. This might entail planning for transportation to and from the hospital, as well as making changes to your house to fit your rehabilitation requirements. Simple changes, such as putting handrails in the bathroom or fixing loose rugs, may help avoid falls and make it simpler to manage your house safely throughout the recovery period.

Making these lifestyle changes and actively engaging in pre-operative preparations such as physical therapy and exercise will help you get the best possible result after knee replacement surgery. Taking a proactive approach to your health and well-being not only increases the procedure's success but also prepares you for a smoother and more pleasant recovery.

CHAPTER 4

Types Of Knee Replacement Surgery

Total Knee Replacement (TKR)

Total knee replacement surgery, often known as TKR, is a technique used to relieve severe knee pain and restore function in individuals with advanced arthritis or major knee injury. During a TKR, the surgeon removes diseased cartilage and bone from the knee joint and replaces it with prosthetic metal and plastic components.

The process starts with the patient being given an anesthetic to enhance comfort and reduce discomfort during surgery. After the anesthetic has taken effect, the surgeon makes an incision above the knee to expose the joint. The injured surfaces of the femur (thigh bone) and tibia (shin bone) are then meticulously removed using precision equipment.

The surgeon then molds the leftover bone to fit the prosthetic knee components. A metal implant is affixed to the femur's end, and a plastic implant is fastened to the tibia's top. These components mirror the knee joint's natural structure and function.

Furthermore, if the bottom of the kneecap is injured, a plastic button may be affixed to the rear of the kneecap to provide a smooth surface for movement. Once all of the components are in place, the incision is closed and the patient is sent to a recovery area.

Patients often receive physical therapy after surgery to recover knee strength and range of motion. With careful rehabilitation and attention to post-operative instructions, many patients report considerable pain and mobility improvement after TKR.

Partial Knee Replacement (PKR)

Partial knee replacement, also known as unicompartmental knee replacement, is a surgical treatment that targets specific regions of deterioration inside the knee joint. Unlike total knee replacement, which replaces the complete knee joint, PKR focuses on the damaged area of the knee while conserving healthy tissue and bone if feasible.

The treatment starts with the physician creating a smaller incision than TKR, usually on the side of the knee. This enables focused access to the injured compartment of the knee joint while preserving the undamaged portions. Once the joint has been exposed, the surgeon will remove the diseased cartilage and bone from the afflicted compartment.

The surgeon will next implant prosthetic components that are carefully engineered to suit the knee's remaining healthy surfaces. These components may consist of a metal implant for the femur and a plastic implant for the tibia, comparable to those used in TKR but on a smaller size.

Because PKR is less intrusive than TKR and retains more of the original knee architecture, it often leads to quicker recovery periods and less post-operative discomfort. However, not all patients are eligible for PKR, which is most successful in individuals with isolated knee arthritis or injury to a single compartment of the knee.

Revision Knee Replacement

Revision knee replacement is a surgical technique that replaces a defective or damaged knee implant following a prior knee replacement operation. While the majority of knee replacements are successful, issues such as implant loosening, infection, or wear and tear over time may need revision surgery.

The technique is identical to primary knee replacement, but it may provide extra issues because of scar tissue, bone loss, or other complications from the previous operation. The surgeon carefully removes the current implants, repairs any bone or soft tissue damage, and then replaces the components with new implants.

To obtain the best results, revision knee replacement must be carefully planned and performed using specialist surgical procedures. In certain circumstances, the surgeon may need to utilize specialist implants or bone transplants to repair bone loss or instability.

Because of the intricacy of the treatment and the possibility of further therapy, recovery from revision knee replacement may take longer and be more difficult than following the first knee replacement. However, for patients who have prolonged discomfort or instability after an initial knee replacement, revision surgery might provide fresh hope for greater function and quality of life.

Minimally Invasive Knee Replacement Techniques

Minimally invasive knee replacement treatments strive to lessen the size of the incision and the stress on surrounding tissues when compared to typical knee replacement surgeries. While the procedure's aims remain the same (pain relief and function restoration), the surgical method and tools change.

During minimally invasive knee replacement, the surgeon creates a smaller incision and typically employs specialized devices and procedures to get access to the knee joint. This may include the use of arthroscopy, a minimally invasive surgical method that visualizes and treats the joint using a tiny camera and small equipment placed via small incisions.

Minimally invasive knee replacement procedures, which minimize tissue disturbance and stress, may result in shorter recovery periods, less post-operative discomfort, and better esthetic results than standard open surgery. However, not all patients are candidates for minimally invasive procedures, and the choice to adopt this strategy is based on the patient's anatomy, the degree of the knee injury, and the surgeon's experience.

Overall, minimally invasive knee replacement is a promising alternative for patients looking for a less intrusive approach to knee replacement surgery, with the potential for faster recovery and better results. However, it is critical to contact a trained orthopedic surgeon to identify the best treatment approach based on your specific requirements and situation.

CHAPTER 5

The Surgical

Anesthesia Options

Anesthesia is essential for a painless and pleasant knee replacement operation. There are commonly three types of anesthesia: general anesthesia, regional anesthesia, and a combination of the two.

1. General Anesthesia: With this option, you will be entirely asleep throughout the procedure. It entails delivering drugs via an IV or inhalation to produce sleep and alleviate discomfort. This is often favored for people who have difficulties laying motionless or are having more sophisticated treatments.

2. Regional anesthesia, as opposed to general anesthesia, numbs the area around the knee by targeting particular nerves. Common forms include spinal and epidural anesthesia.

With this method, you will be awake throughout the procedure but will not experience any discomfort in the affected region. It also has fewer adverse effects than general anesthesia.

3. Mixture anesthetic: Sometimes a mixture of general and regional anesthetic is employed. For example, general anesthesia may be used to induce drowsiness before switching to a regional anesthetic to keep discomfort at bay during surgery. This strategy combines the advantages of both solutions while reducing their respective downsides.

The choice of anesthetic is determined by several criteria, including your general health, preferences, and the surgeon's advice. Your anesthesiologist will work closely with you to establish the best solution for your condition.

Step-By-Step Overview Of Surgery

Understanding the step-by-step process of knee replacement surgery might help to reduce anxiety about the treatment.

While the precise processes may vary significantly based on the surgical method utilized and any individual patient considerations, the following is a basic overview:

1. **Preparation:** Before the procedure, you will be transported to the operating room and placed on the operating table. The surgical team will clean and sterilize the region surrounding your knee.

2. **Incision:** The surgeon will create an incision above the knee, usually along the front or side. The size of the incision may vary, with less invasive procedures often necessitating smaller ones.

3. **Resection of Damaged Tissues:** Once the knee joint has been exposed, the surgeon will gently remove the

damaged cartilage and bone from the thighbone (femur) and shinbone (tibia). This makes room for the prosthetic components.

4. Implant Placement: The artificial components, which include metal implants for the femur and tibia, as well as a plastic spacer for the gap in between, are firmly installed. These components are typically cemented in place, however cementless procedures are also available.

5. Closure: After checking the implants' appropriate placement and alignment, the surgeon will stitch or staple the incision. A sterile dressing is subsequently put on the wound.

Duration Of Surgery

The time of knee replacement surgery varies based on several variables, including the procedure's complexity, the patient's general health, and the surgical method employed. On average, the procedure lasts between one and two hours.

Minimally invasive procedures, which use smaller incisions and minimal tissue damage, may result in shorter operative timeframes than standard open surgery. To get the best results, accuracy, and thoroughness must be prioritized above speed.

Potential Risks And Complications

While knee replacement surgery is typically safe and successful, it does include certain risks and problems, as with any surgical operation. It is important to be aware of these dangers and address them with your physician beforehand. Some common hazards are:

1. **Infection:** Even with careful sterile methods, there is a danger of developing an infection at the surgery site. This danger may be reduced with medicines and adequate wound care.

2. Blood Clots: Surgery and subsequent immobilization may raise the risk of developing blood clots in the legs (deep vein thrombosis) or lungs (pulmonary embolism). Blood thinners and early mobilization are two measures that may help lessen this danger.

3. Implant Problems: While rare, complications like implant loosening, dislocation, or wear and tear over time may occur. Regular follow-up meetings with your surgeon may help discover and treat possible problems early on.

4. Nerve or Blood Vessel Damage: During surgery, there is a small chance of injuring surrounding nerves or blood vessels, which may cause numbness, weakness, or bleeding. However, skilled surgeons make efforts to reduce the danger.

5. Allergic Reactions or Anesthesia difficulties: In rare cases, individuals may develop allergic reactions to drugs or difficulties from anesthesia.

Your medical staff will continuously monitor you during the procedure to treat any issues that arise.

By recognizing the possible risks and problems and taking the necessary measures, you may approach knee replacement surgery with confidence and peace of mind.

CHAPTER 6

Recovery Process

The Hospital Stay After Surgery

Following knee replacement surgery, patients are often admitted to the hospital for a few days to ensure adequate monitoring and healing. During this period, medical personnel will continuously check vital signs, treat pain, provide medicines, and aid with movement.

When patients wake up following surgery, they are usually sent to a recovery room where medical personnel examine their status and ensure that there are no immediate issues. Once stabilized, patients are transported to a hospital room to begin their recuperation.

Throughout the hospital stay, nurses and physical therapists will help patients get out of bed, walk using support equipment like crutches or walkers, and do basic exercises to improve blood circulation and avoid stiffness.

Pain Management Strategies

Effective pain management is critical for a successful recovery after knee replacement surgery. To relieve discomfort during the early healing phase, doctors usually prescribe a mix of pain drugs. Nonsteroidal anti-inflammatory medicines (NSAIDs), opioid medications, and local anesthesia procedures may all be used.

In addition to medicine, various pain relief treatments may be used, such as cold therapy, leg elevation, and relaxation techniques. Ice packs may decrease swelling and numb the region surrounding the surgery site, relieving discomfort. Elevating the leg above the level of the heart may help to minimize swelling and pain.

Furthermore, relaxation methods such as deep breathing exercises, guided visualization, and meditation may help patients avoid discomfort and foster a feeling of calm and well-being throughout their recovery.

Physical Therapy And Rehabilitation Exercises

Physical therapy is essential in the rehabilitation process after knee replacement surgery. Patients usually begin mild exercises to enhance strength, flexibility, and range of motion in the knee joint shortly after surgery, guided by a physical therapist.

Initially, workouts may include basic motions like ankle pumps, quadriceps sets, and moderate knee bends. As the patient's condition improves, more complex workouts including leg lifts, hamstring stretches, and stationary cycling may be added.

Physical therapy sessions may take place both in the hospital and on an outpatient basis after release. The number and intensity of treatment sessions will vary according to the patient's development and general health.

Expected Recovery Timeline

The recovery period following knee replacement surgery varies based on several variables, including the patient's age, general health, and the scope of the operation. However, a basic chronology might help patients understand what to anticipate throughout their recuperation.

Patients usually suffer some pain and discomfort in the days after surgery, which progressively improves over the next several weeks. By the end of the first month, many patients can accomplish basic daily tasks with little help.

By the third month after surgery, most patients have made good progress in their rehabilitation and may participate in more rigorous activities, such as walking longer distances and climbing stairs more easily.

However, patients may need to wait six months to a year to see the greatest improvement in strength, mobility, and function.

Throughout the healing process, patients must follow their healthcare provider's recommendations, attend physical therapy sessions regularly, and show patience and tenacity as they seek to restore full knee joint function.

CHAPTER 7

Post-Op Care

Homecare Instructions

Following knee replacement surgery, it is critical to follow particular home care guidelines to promote adequate healing and a full recovery. Your healthcare team will give extensive instructions geared to your unique circumstances; nonetheless, here are some broad pointers to remember:

1. Activity Level: While progressively increasing your activity level is necessary for regaining strength and mobility, it is also critical to prevent over-exertion. Follow your surgeon's instructions for weight-bearing limitations and physical therapy exercises. Begin with modest motions and progressively increase as acceptable.

2. Pain Management: It is typical to have discomfort or pain after surgery. Your doctor will prescribe pain medicines to ease your discomfort. Take them exactly as prescribed, and notify your doctor right away if you have any unexpected discomfort or side effects.

3. Mobility Aids: Depending on your condition and surgical method, you may need mobility aids such as crutches, a walker, or a cane to help you move during the early recovery phase. Use these tools as directed by your healthcare provider to help avoid falls and support your recovering knee.

4. Diet & Nutrition: A well-balanced, nutrient-dense diet is crucial for facilitating healing and general health. Ensure that you are receiving enough protein, vitamins, and minerals to help tissue regeneration and recovery. Maintain hydration by drinking lots of water throughout the day.

5. Follow-Up Appointments: Make every planned follow-up visit with your surgeon and physical therapist.

These visits are critical for tracking your progress, resolving any concerns or issues, and changing your treatment plan as necessary.

6. Home Environment: Make changes to your living environment to facilitate a safe and pleasant recuperation. Remove any impediments or dangers that might cause trips or falls, build handrails in corridors and bathrooms, and consider utilizing assistive equipment like a raised toilet seat or shower chair to help with everyday tasks.

By carefully following these home care guidelines, you may promote optimum healing, reduce problems, and achieve the best possible result after knee replacement surgery.

Wound Care

Proper wound care is critical for avoiding infection and encouraging recovery after knee replacement surgery. Your healthcare team will provide you with specific advice depending on your unique situation, but here are some broad suggestions to follow:

1. Keep the Incision Clean and Dry: To avoid infection, the surgical incision should be kept clean and dry. Follow your surgeon's instructions for when to remove the dressing and how to clean the incision site. Cleanse the area with gentle soap and water, then pat it dry with a clean towel.

2. Change Dressings as Directed: Your surgeon may prescribe that you change the dressing over the incision site frequently. Follow their directions for dressing changes and the kind of dressing to use. If you see any indications of infection, such as increased redness, swelling, or discharge from the incision, call your healthcare professional right away.

3. Monitor for Infection: Keep an eye on the incision site for any symptoms of infection, such as redness, warmth, swelling, or yellow, green, or odorous discharge. Also, keep an eye out for fever or chills, which might be signs of an infection. If you encounter any of these symptoms, please inform your doctor right away.

4. Prevent Irritating the Incision: Use caution around the incision site to prevent irritating or disturbing the healing tissue. Avoid activities that may put pressure on the incision, such as heavy bending or twisting, and do not soak in baths or swim until your surgeon has cleared you.

5. Follow-Up Care: Attend all planned follow-up consultations with your surgeon to check the healing of your incision. Your surgeon may remove stitches or staples as required and evaluate the general condition of your knee replacement.

By adhering to these wound care instructions and swiftly addressing any concerns or issues, you may help the healing process and lower your risk of complications after knee replacement surgery.

Medication Management

Medication management is an integral part of post-operative treatment after knee replacement surgery. Your healthcare team will prescribe drugs to alleviate pain, prevent infection, and lower the risk of blood clots. Here are some important considerations to bear in mind:

1. **Pain Management:** To help you feel better after surgery, your doctor will prescribe pain medicines. Take these drugs exactly as suggested, and don't wait until the pain is severe before taking them. Staying ahead of the pain is critical for your comfort and mobility throughout the healing process.

2. **Antibiotics:** To avoid infection, your surgeon may prescribe antibiotics to be taken after surgery. It is critical to take these drugs precisely as recommended and complete the whole course, even if you begin to feel better before the treatment is done.

3. Blood Thinners: Knee replacement surgery raises the danger of blood clots developing in your legs (deep vein thrombosis) or migrating to your lungs (pulmonary embolism). To lower this risk, your doctor may give blood thinners or suggest additional precautions such as compression stockings or leg exercises.

4. Other drugs: In addition to pain relievers, antibiotics, and blood thinners, you may be taking drugs to treat pre-existing diseases including high blood pressure or diabetes. Continue to take these drugs as prescribed, unless otherwise ordered by your healthcare practitioner.

5. Side Effects: Be aware of any possible side effects linked with your drugs, and report any odd symptoms or reactions to your healthcare professional right away. Symptoms include nausea, vomiting, disorientation, and allergic responses.

6. Medication Schedule: Keep track of your medication schedule to verify that you are taking the proper meds at the appropriate times. Keep track of your meds using pill organizers or smartphone applications.

You may decrease pain, lower the risk of problems, and encourage a successful recovery after knee replacement surgery by managing your medicines efficiently and following your healthcare provider's recommendations.

Monitoring For Complications

While knee replacement surgery is typically safe and successful, it is critical to monitor for any issues throughout the recovery period. Here are some frequent difficulties to look for:

1. Infection: Surgical site infections may arise after knee replacement surgery. Look for indications of infection, such as increased redness, edema, temperature, or discharge from the incision site.

Also, keep an eye out for fever or chills, which might be signs of an infection. If you encounter any of these symptoms, you should contact your doctor immediately.

2. Blood Clots: Knee replacement surgery raises the danger of blood clots developing in your legs (deep vein thrombosis) or migrating to your lungs (pulmonary embolism). Be aware of signs such as swelling, soreness, warmth, or redness in your legs, as well as chest pain or trouble breathing. If you suffer any of these symptoms, get medical treatment immediately.

3. Joint Stiffness or Instability: While some degree of stiffness and instability in the knee joint is typical after surgery, severe or increasing symptoms may signal a problem. If you notice any substantial changes in your range of motion, strength, or stability, notify your healthcare physician.

4. Nerve Damage: Nerve damage is an uncommon but possible side effect of knee replacement surgery. Look for symptoms including numbness, tingling, or weakness in the afflicted limb, as well as changes in sensation or motor function.

CHAPTER 8

Lifestyle Modifications Following Surgery

Adaptive Equipment And Aids

Adapting to life after knee replacement surgery sometimes entails altering your daily routine and surroundings. Adaptive devices and assistance are critical to enabling this shift. These items are intended to help you accomplish daily chores with increased ease and comfort while safeguarding your recently replaced knee.

A walker or cane is an important piece of adapted equipment that offers stability and support when walking. These devices assist in shifting your weight away from your knee joint, decreasing strain, and avoiding falls. Furthermore, installing grab bars in your bathroom and handrails along stairs may give additional support and help to avoid accidents.

Other adapted equipment includes elevated toilet seats, shower chairs, and long-handled reachers, which reduce the need for excessive bending or reaching. These gadgets reduce stress on your knee joint while also promoting freedom throughout regular tasks.

Recommended Exercises To Strengthen The Knee

Physical therapy is essential in the recovery process after knee replacement surgery. The recommended exercises strengthen the muscles around the knee joint, improve flexibility, and increase general mobility.

Initially, workouts may include modest motions to develop a range of motion and reduce stiffness. Your physical therapist will gradually introduce increasingly demanding activities to help you gain strength and endurance. Leg lifts, knee extensions, and hamstring curls may all be performed using resistance bands or weights.

Another excellent method for strengthening the knee joint without putting it under excessive stress is aquatic treatment, which is conducted in a pool. Water's buoyancy decreases pressure on your joints while providing resistance to help you build muscular strength and flexibility.

Exercises after surgery need consistency. Following an organized workout routine will help you heal faster and restore the full function of your knee.

Dietary Concerns For Optimal Recovery

Nutrition is critical for maintaining good recovery after knee replacement surgery. A well-balanced diet high in key nutrients helps decrease inflammation, promote tissue healing, and strengthen bones.

Consume protein-rich meals, such as lean meats, fish, eggs, and lentils, to help in muscle regeneration and recovery. Incorporate lots of fruits and vegetables, which are high in vitamins, minerals, and antioxidants that stimulate tissue mending and immunological function.

Omega-3 fatty acids, found in fatty fish such as salmon and walnuts, have anti-inflammatory qualities that may aid with postoperative pain and edema. Additionally, proper hydration is essential for joint lubrication and general health, so drink lots of water throughout the day.

Avoiding excessive alcohol intake and sugary, processed meals will help you recover faster. Consulting with a licensed dietitian may assist you in creating a customized nutrition plan based on your requirements and objectives.

Return To Daily Activities And Work

Gradually returning to your normal activities and job routine is a crucial part of the rehabilitation process after knee replacement surgery. While it's important to listen to your body and prevent overexertion, being active and involved may help you recover quicker and feel better overall.

Begin by gradually increasing the time and intensity of your activities, concentrating on low-impact exercises that are easy on your knee joint. Walking, swimming, and cycling are good ways to increase endurance and strength without putting undue strain on your knee.

When you return to work, consider modifying your workspace to meet your requirements. This may involve using an ergonomic chair, altering the height of your desk, or taking regular pauses to relax and stretch your legs.

Communicate honestly with your healthcare team and employer about any concerns or limits you may have when you return to work. They may provide assistance and direction to enable a seamless and successful return to your usual routine.

By making these lifestyle changes and integrating prescribed exercises, nutritional considerations, and techniques for returning to everyday activities and work, you may maximize your recovery and reap the advantages of your knee replacement surgery for years to come.

CHAPTER 9

Possible Complications And Risks

Infection is one of the most serious consequences of knee replacement surgery. Despite extensive sterility procedures in the operating area, there is always the potential for bacterial contamination, which may lead to infection. This danger exists even after surgery, since germs may enter the body via a variety of routes, including the incision site and the bloodstream.

Early indicators of infection may include increasing pain, edema, warmth, redness, or discharge from the surgical site. In certain situations, fever and chills may also develop. Early detection and treatment of infection are critical for preventing its spread and possible harm to the replacement knee joint.

Antibiotics are often used to treat infections, either orally or intravenously, depending on their severity. In more severe situations, surgical intervention may be required to remove contaminated tissue or replace the prosthetic joint.

Preventive methods include rigorous preoperative screening for any existing infections, strict adherence to sterile practices during surgery, and postoperative measures including antibiotic prophylaxis and wound care.

Blood Clots

Blood clots, commonly known as deep vein thrombosis (DVT), are another major danger of knee replacement surgery. This happens when blood clots develop in the deep veins of the legs, usually as a result of restricted movement and blood flow during the healing phase.

DVT symptoms might include discomfort, edema, warmth, and redness in the afflicted limb. However, it is important to remember that not all blood clots produce symptoms, making identification difficult.

If left untreated, blood clots may break free and migrate to the lungs, resulting in a potentially fatal illness known as pulmonary embolism. A pulmonary embolism may cause abrupt shortness of breath, chest discomfort, a fast pulse rate, and a bloody cough.

Early mobilization, compression stockings, pneumatic compression devices, and blood-thinning drugs like heparin or aspirin are all preventive methods to lower the risk of blood clotting. These measures are intended to enhance circulation and avoid the development of blood clots during the healing phase.

Implant Failure

Implant failure, albeit uncommon, is a significant complication that may occur after knee replacement surgery. This may happen for several reasons, including mechanical difficulties with the implant components, incorrect placement after surgery, or poor bone quality.

Implant failure symptoms may include chronic discomfort, instability, restricted range of motion, and trouble bearing weight on the afflicted knee. In certain circumstances, patients may notice audible disturbances coming from the joint, such as clicking or squeaking.

When implant failure is suspected, diagnostic imaging procedures like as X-rays or MRI scans may be used to determine the artificial joint's integrity. Treatment options vary depending on the underlying reason, ranging from conservative methods like physical therapy to revision surgery to replace the damaged implant.

To reduce the risk of implant failure, surgeons carefully examine their patients' anatomy, choose suitable implant components, and guarantee correct placement during surgery. Furthermore, following postoperative rehabilitation procedures and sticking to weight-bearing limitations might aid improve long-term results.

Nerve Or Blood Vessel Damage

Nerve or blood vessel injury is a possible consequence of knee replacement surgery, although it is rare. During the surgery, neighboring nerves and blood arteries may be mistakenly injured as a result of surgical manipulation or trauma.

Nerve injury symptoms might include numbness, tingling, weakness, or alterations in feeling in the afflicted leg or foot. In contrast, symptoms of vascular damage in the afflicted limb may include edema, redness, or a decreased pulse.

Early detection of nerve or blood vessel injury is crucial in avoiding long-term problems. In some circumstances, conservative treatment such as physical therapy or medication may be sufficient to alleviate symptoms. However, severe or chronic instances may need surgical intervention to repair or rebuild damaged structures.

Surgeons take steps to reduce the risk of nerve and blood vascular damage during knee replacement surgery by carefully identifying and safeguarding these structures. Patients are also informed about probable signs and symptoms so that they may report them to their healthcare professionals for proper examination and treatment.

CHAPTER 10

Long-Term Prospects And Follow-Up

Longevity Of Knee Implants

Knee replacement surgery is an important step in improving the quality of life for those suffering from crippling knee pain and restricted mobility. One of the primary worries that patients have is the lifetime of the implants utilized after surgery. Understanding the elements that determine the lifetime of knee implants may help patients make educated selections and manage their expectations.

Modern knee implants are designed to survive for 15 years or more. However, the longevity of an implant varies based on several variables, including the patient's age, activity level, weight, general health, and implant type. Implant lifetime may be an issue for younger and more active individuals, since physical activity may place additional strain on the implant.

Material and technological advancements have greatly enhanced the longevity of knee implants. Materials like titanium and ceramic are recognized for their strength and resistance to wear, which helps the implants last longer. Furthermore, advances in surgical methods, such as minimally invasive procedures, may extend the life of knee implants by lowering tissue damage and the risk of problems.

Regular follow-up meetings with the surgeon are required to check the quality of the implants and discover any symptoms of wear and tear early on. X-rays and other imaging tests may be done to evaluate the implants' integrity and detect any problems that need action.

Monitoring For Signs Of Wear And Tear

After knee replacement surgery, patients must monitor their implants for symptoms of wear and tear. While contemporary knee implants are intended to be long-lasting, they are nonetheless susceptible to deterioration over time, particularly with high levels of physical activity or severe stress on the joint.

Common indicators of wear and tear on knee implants include chronic discomfort, swelling, instability, stiffness, or a reduction in range of motion. These symptoms may appear gradually over time and might signal implant loosening, wear, or other difficulties.

In addition to monitoring for physical symptoms, patients should be aware of any changes in their activity level or lifestyle that might affect the lifespan of their implants. High-impact sports and carrying extra weight may increase wear and tear on knee implants, thereby shortening their lifetime.

Regular follow-up meetings with the surgeon are required to check the quality of the implants and discover any symptoms of wear and tear early on. During these visits, the surgeon may do physical exams, examine imaging studies, and address any concerns or changes in symptoms with the patient.

Follow-Up Appointments With The Surgeon

Following knee replacement surgery, patients are usually scheduled for frequent follow-up consultations with their surgeon to monitor their recovery and evaluate the status of their implants. These follow-up consultations are critical for maintaining optimum results and spotting issues early on.

During follow-up visits, the surgeon will do a complete physical examination of the knee to look for evidence of healing, range of motion, and stability. X-rays or other imaging tests may be conducted to determine the location and condition of the implants.

Patients should utilize follow-up sessions to address any concerns or changes in symptoms. Open communication with the surgeon is vital, as is providing thorough information regarding any discomfort, edema, or functional limits.

In addition to physical exams and imaging testing, follow-up meetings may include talks regarding rehabilitation exercises, activity adjustments, and methods for preserving knee health after surgery. The surgeon may advice on how to gradually raise activity levels, avoid high-impact activities, and preserve the knee joint from undue stress.

Tips For Maintaining Knee Health After Surgery

After knee replacement surgery, patients must make proactive efforts to ensure the health and durability of their new knee joint. While contemporary knee implants are built to last, patients may do a few things to limit wear and tear and the risk of problems.

1. Follow Rehabilitation Guidelines: Participating in a complete rehabilitation program is critical for facilitating healing, regaining strength and flexibility, and improving functional results. Patients should attentively adhere to the exercises and directions given by their physical therapist or healthcare team.

2. Maintain a Healthy Weight: Excess weight may place additional strain on the knee joint, increasing the likelihood of implant deterioration and problems. Maintaining a healthy weight with a balanced diet and regular exercise may help prevent knee strain and improve overall joint health.

3. Stay Active: While high-impact activities may be avoided following knee replacement surgery, keeping active is still essential for joint mobility, muscular strength, and cardiovascular health. Low-impact activities like walking, swimming, and cycling are often advised.

4. Avoid Overexertion: Activities like heavy lifting, jogging, and leaping may place too much pressure on the knee joint. Instead, concentrate on tasks that are easy on the joints and can be done without difficulty or suffering.

5. Protect the Knee Joint: To ensure the knee joint's long-term health, take care to keep it safe from harm. This may include wearing supportive footwear, utilizing assistance equipment such as canes or braces as required, and avoiding uneven or slippery surfaces.

By following these guidelines and being proactive about knee health after surgery, patients may help guarantee the long-term success of their knee replacement and enjoy enhanced mobility and quality of life for years to come. Regular follow-up meetings with the surgeon, as well as open discussion about any concerns or changes in symptoms, are also required for early detection and resolution of any difficulties.

Conclusion

To summarize, knee replacement surgery is a light of hope for those suffering from excruciating knee pain and reduced mobility caused by illnesses such as osteoarthritis, rheumatoid arthritis, or accidents. Through this detailed guide, we've gone into the various nuances of this transformational operation, to provide clear knowledge to people considering or undergoing it.

First, we looked at the structure of the knee joint, determining its critical function in enabling mobility and weight-bearing tasks. Understanding the anatomy and function of the knee lays the groundwork for understanding why problems requiring knee replacement surgery may have a significant effect on one's quality of life.

We then went through the diagnostic process, from detecting symptoms to conducting testing such as X-rays and MRIs. A timely and correct diagnosis is critical in assessing the need and feasibility of knee replacement surgery, ensuring that patients get appropriate therapy based on their situation.

This book also discussed several conservative therapy methods for controlling knee pain and increasing joint function before surgery. Medication, physical therapy, lifestyle changes, and assistive technologies are all possible options. While these procedures may give comfort to some, others may find that their disease worsens to the point where surgical surgery is the only realistic choice.

The surgical procedure was explained in detail, beginning with pre-operative preparations and ending with post-operative care. Surgical advances, such as minimally invasive methods and robotic-assisted surgery, have improved the accuracy and outcomes of knee replacement treatments, resulting in quicker recovery periods and better long-term outcomes.

Furthermore, we investigated the possible dangers and consequences of knee replacement surgery, highlighting the significance of informed consent and detailed talks with healthcare practitioners to reduce these risks.

Finally, we emphasized the importance of post-operative rehabilitation in improving the outcome of knee replacement surgery. Rehabilitation is critical in restoring strength, flexibility, and function to the knee joint, enabling people to recover independence and resume normal activities.

In essence, knee replacement surgery is a multidisciplinary strategy intended to relieve pain, restore function, and improve the quality of life for those suffering from severe knee joint disorders. This handbook is a great resource for navigating the complexity of knee replacement surgery, supporting informed decision-making and best results for both patients and healthcare professionals.

THE END

www.ingramcontent.com/pod-product-compliance
Lightning Source LLC
Chambersburg PA
CBHW061253250726
48653CB00002B/640